Ashes & Valor: The Story of Firefighting Through The Ages

Firefighting is the act of extinguishing fires and protecting lives and property from the devastation of flames. It is a critical public service that has saved countless lives and prevented immeasurable damage to buildings, homes, and other structures.

The history of firefighting dates back to ancient times, when communities would band together to fight fires with rudimentary tools such as water, sand, and animal skins. Over time, firefighting techniques and equipment have evolved, leading to the creation of professional fire departments and advanced technologies that have made firefighting safer and more effective.

In this extensive history of firefighting, we will explore the fascinating and often humorous history of this essential service, paying tribute to the brave firefighters who put their lives on the line to protect others. From the ancient world to the modern era, we will examine the evolution of firefighting and the impact it has had on societies around the world.

Ancient Origins

The history of firefighting can be traced back to ancient civilizations, where communities developed basic techniques to fight fires. In ancient Egypt, for example, citizens used buckets and jars to carry water from the Nile River to extinguish fires. In Greece, citizens used a siphon-like device called a syringe to pump water from a container and spray it on flames.

In ancient Rome, the city's fire brigades consisted of slaves and criminals who were forced to fight fires as part of their punishment. They used tools such as hooks, buckets, and axes to contain and extinguish fires.

In China, the use of gunpowder and explosives were sometimes used to create firebreaks to stop the spread of fires. In Japan, bamboo ladders and buckets of water were used to fight fires in wooden buildings.

Although ancient firefighting techniques were crude by modern standards, they laid the foundation for future developments in firefighting technology and techniques. The lessons learned from these early efforts to fight fires would be invaluable in the centuries to come.

During the Middle Ages, the rise of cities and towns led to an increased risk of fires, as buildings were often constructed from highly flammable materials such as wood and thatch. As a result, firefighting became a more organized and professional endeavor during this period.

In Europe, firefighting guilds and religious orders were established to provide firefighting services to cities and towns. These groups were responsible for creating bucket brigades, using hand-operated pumps, and developing techniques to prevent fires from spreading. Some of the earliest fire insurance companies were also established during this time, allowing property owners to protect their investments against the risk of fire.

Despite these advancements, the lack of water sources and adequate firefighting equipment continued to pose challenges. In many cases, entire towns and cities were devastated by fires that could not be contained. One of the most notable fires of this era was the Great Fire of London in 1666, which destroyed much of the city and led to the development of more advanced firefighting techniques and technologies.

The advent of the Industrial Revolution brought significant changes to firefighting in the 18th and 19th centuries. New technologies such as steam engines and iron pipes allowed for more effective water delivery to fires, while the introduction of fire-resistant materials such as concrete and steel made buildings less susceptible to fires.

Professional fire departments also began to emerge during this time, with the first one established in Edinburgh, Scotland in 1824. These departments were staffed by trained firefighters who were equipped with more advanced tools and equipment, such as hoses, nozzles, and hydrants.

In the United States, volunteer fire companies were prevalent in many cities and towns, with volunteers often competing with one another to see who could respond to fires the fastest. These companies were eventually replaced by paid fire departments, which were better equipped to handle the increasing number of fires that were occurring in urban areas.

Despite these advancements, firefighting was still a dangerous and often deadly profession. Firefighters continued to face significant risks from smoke inhalation, burns, and collapsing buildings. Nonetheless, their bravery and dedication to saving lives and property was lauded by communities across the globe.

The 20th century saw significant advancements in firefighting technology and techniques. The widespread adoption of motorized fire trucks and aerial ladders allowed firefighters to access previously inaccessible areas, while the development of breathing apparatus and fire-resistant gear made firefighting less dangerous for those on the front lines.

The Impact of world wars on firefighting was significant, with firefighters playing a crucial role in both war efforts. In addition to fighting fires caused by enemy bombing campaigns, firefighters were also instrumental in rescuing civilians and soldiers from burning buildings and other hazardous situations.

The rise of volunteer firefighting continued in the 20th century, with many communities relying on volunteer fire departments to provide firefighting services. The use of technology, such as thermal imaging cameras and communication systems, has also allowed firefighters to better locate and extinguish fires.

National firefighting standards and organizations were also established during this time, allowing for greater coordination and cooperation among firefighters around the world. The dedication and sacrifices of firefighters continued to be lauded by communities and governments alike, with firefighters being recognized as some of the bravest and most selfless public servants.

Throughout history, firefighters have been honored and recognized for their bravery and dedication to protecting their communities. In many cultures, firefighters are considered heroes, and their sacrifices are celebrated through various traditions and rituals.

Firefighting badges and medals are often awarded to firefighters for their service and bravery. In some communities, firefighters are given the honor of carrying the flag at local events, while in others, they are invited to lead parades and processions.

In addition to formal recognition, firefighters are also supported by their communities in more informal ways. For example, many firehouses have been adopted by local businesses and organizations, who provide donations and support to the firefighters who work there. Fundraisers and charity events are also often held to raise money for firefighting equipment and other needs.

The sacrifices that firefighters make on a daily basis are immeasurable, and communities around the world owe a debt of gratitude to these brave men and women. By honoring their service and supporting their efforts, we can ensure that firefighting remains a vital and essential public service for generations to come.

The Evolution of Firefighting

Firefighting dates back to ancient times, where communities developed basic techniques to fight fires. Early civilizations such as Egypt, Rome, Greece, and China all had their own methods of firefighting.

In ancient Egypt, citizens used buckets and jars to carry water from the Nile River to extinguish fires. They also used hand-operated pumps to draw water from wells and pools. Ancient Egyptians also developed a type of fire extinguisher made of clay pots filled with a mixture of water, salt, and vinegar that could be thrown onto small fires.

In Greece, citizens used a siphon-like device called a syringe to pump water from a container and spray it on flames.

Firefighting has been a concern for human communities since ancient times, and early civilizations developed their own methods to fight fires.

In ancient Egypt, people used a bucket and jar brigade to carry water from the Nile River or other sources to extinguish fires. They also employed hand-operated pumps, which were used to draw water from wells and pools. Ancient Egyptians also developed a type of fire extinguisher made of clay pots filled with a mixture of water, salt, and vinegar that could be thrown onto small fires to smother them.

In Greece, the early methods of firefighting involved a siphon-like device called a syringe, which was used to pump water from a container and spray it on flames. The Greeks also developed a water-delivery system that used pipes to carry water from nearby sources to where it was needed most.

In Rome, firefighting was initially performed by slaves and criminals who were forced to fight fires as part of their punishment. They used tools such as hooks, buckets, and axes to contain and extinguish fires. Later, the Roman government established the Vigiles, a firefighting brigade that was made up of 7,000 men who were trained in firefighting techniques.

In China, citizens used several methods to fight fires, including using gunpowder and explosives to create firebreaks to stop the spread of fires. They also used bamboo ladders and buckets of water to fight fires in wooden buildings.

The first organized fire brigades were established in ancient Rome and China, but the idea of a professional firefighting force would not develop until much later. Nonetheless, the lessons learned from these early firefighting methods laid the foundation for future developments in firefighting technology and techniques.

Water has always played a critical role in firefighting, as it is the most effective substance for extinguishing fires. Early methods of firefighting relied heavily on water, and it continues to be the primary tool used to fight fires today.

One of the earliest methods of using water to fight fires was through the use of bucket brigades. In this method, people would form a line and pass buckets of water from one person to the next until it reached the site of the fire. This method was limited by the distance the bucket brigade could reach and the amount of water that could be carried in a single bucket.

As firefighting techniques evolved, so too did the methods for delivering water to fires. Hand-operated pumps were developed, allowing firefighters to draw water from nearby sources and pump it onto flames. Later, motorized fire engines were developed, allowing firefighters to pump large amounts of water from hydrants and other sources directly onto the fire.

In addition to water, other substances have been developed to assist in firefighting. Chemicals such as foams and powders are often used to smother fires, and gases such as carbon dioxide and halon are used to starve fires of oxygen. Nonetheless, water remains the most effective and widely used substance in firefighting to this day.

The first fire brigades emerged in ancient Rome and China, but they were not professional organizations in the modern sense. These brigades were made up of volunteers who would respond to fires and try to contain them using rudimentary tools and techniques.

In Rome, the Vigiles were established in the 1st century AD. This firefighting brigade was made up of around 7,000 men who were responsible for maintaining order in the city and fighting fires. They were divided into seven cohorts, each with its own responsibilities. One cohort was responsible for firefighting, while others were responsible for enforcing building codes and ensuring that the city's water supply was maintained.

In China, the first fire brigade was established in the 5th century BC during the reign of King Wen of Zhou. This brigade was made up of soldiers who were trained to fight fires using bamboo ladders and buckets of water. The Chinese also developed fire extinguishers made of clay pots filled with a mixture of water and vinegar.

During the Middle Ages, firefighting brigades were often established by guilds or religious orders. These brigades were responsible for providing firefighting services to cities and towns and were often made up of volunteers. In some cases, brigades would compete with one another to see who could respond to fires the fastest.

The first professional fire departments did not emerge until the 18th and 19th centuries, with the first one established in Edinburgh, Scotland in 1824. These departments were staffed by trained firefighters who were equipped with more advanced tools and equipment, such as hoses, nozzles, and hydrants. Today, professional fire departments are an essential public service in communities around the world.

In Europe during the Middle Ages, the risk of fires increased as the use of highly flammable materials such as wood and thatch became more prevalent. As a result, firefighting became a more organized and professional endeavor during this period.

Firefighting guilds and religious orders were established to provide firefighting services to cities and towns in Europe. These groups were responsible for creating bucket brigades, using hand-operated pumps, and developing techniques to prevent fires from spreading. Some of the earliest fire insurance companies were also established during this time, allowing property owners to protect their investments against the risk of fire.

Despite these advancements, the lack of water sources and adequate firefighting equipment continued to pose challenges. In many cases, entire towns and cities were devastated by fires that could not be contained. One of the most notable fires of this era was the Great Fire of London in 1666, which destroyed much of the city and led to the development of more advanced firefighting techniques and technologies.

During the 18th and 19th centuries, advancements in technology and firefighting equipment led to the establishment of professional fire departments in many European cities. Despite these advancements, firefighting remained a dangerous and often deadly profession, with firefighters facing significant risks from smoke inhalation, burns, and collapsing buildings. Nonetheless, their bravery and dedication to saving lives and property was lauded by communities across Europe.

The Great Fire of London was one of the most significant fires in European history. The fire started in a baker's shop on Pudding Lane and quickly spread, fueled by strong winds and the use of highly flammable materials in the city's buildings.

Despite efforts to contain the fire, including the use of bucket brigades and firebreaks, the fire continued to spread, ultimately destroying over 13,000 homes and 87 churches. The Royal Exchange and the Bridewell Palace were also destroyed, along with many other important buildings.

The Great Fire of London had a significant impact on firefighting in Europe, leading to the development of more advanced firefighting techniques and technologies. One of the most important developments was the creation of fire insurance companies, which provided property owners with a means of protecting their investments against the risk of fire.

The fire also led to the establishment of fire brigades in London and other European cities. These brigades were equipped with more advanced firefighting tools and equipment, such as hand-operated pumps and fire engines. They were also responsible for enforcing building codes and other regulations to prevent fires from starting in the first place.

Despite these advancements, the Great Fire of London remains a tragic reminder of the devastating impact that fires can have on communities. Nonetheless, the lessons learned from this event continue to inform modern firefighting techniques and technologies, ensuring that firefighters are better equipped than ever to protect lives and property.

Benjamin Franklin was an American statesman, inventor, and scientist who is perhaps best known for his role in drafting the United States Declaration of Independence. However, he also played an important role in the development of firefighting techniques and technologies.

In 1736, Franklin organized the Union Fire Company in Philadelphia, which was the first volunteer firefighting company in the United

States. He also developed several important firefighting innovations, including the first fire insurance company in the United States and a type of fire stove that could be used to heat buildings without creating a fire hazard.

Franklin also developed the first fire engine with a suction hose, which allowed firefighters to draw water from a nearby source and pump it directly onto a fire. This innovation significantly improved the efficiency and effectiveness of firefighting operations.

In addition to his innovations in firefighting technology, Franklin was also a proponent of fire prevention.

He promoted the use of lightning rods on buildings to prevent fires caused by lightning strikes and advocated for the use of building codes to reduce the risk of fires starting in the first place.

Today, Benjamin Franklin is remembered as one of the pioneers of modern firefighting. Firefighters around the world continue to benefit from his innovations and ideas.

The Industrial Revolution, which began in the late 18th century, had a significant impact on firefighting. The increased use of machinery and the concentration of people and industry in urban areas led to an increase in the number and severity of fires.

As a result, new firefighting technologies and techniques were developed to keep pace with the changing landscape. One of the most significant developments was the creation of fire-resistant materials, such as iron and steel, which were used to construct buildings and bridges. This made it more difficult for fires to spread and reduced the risk of catastrophic fires.

The invention of the steam engine also had a significant impact on firefighting. Steam-powered fire engines were faster and more powerful than their hand-operated counterparts, allowing firefighters to respond to fires more quickly and effectively.

Firefighting organizations also became more professional during this time. Many cities and towns established paid fire departments, staffed by trained firefighters who were equipped with the latest firefighting tools and equipment. The use of fire alarms and telegraph systems also improved the speed and efficiency of firefighting operations.

Despite these advancements, fires continued to be a significant problem during the Industrial Revolution. The Great Chicago Fire of 1871, which destroyed much of the city, was a stark reminder of the destructive power of fires. Nonetheless, the lessons learned from these events continue to inform modern firefighting techniques and technologies, ensuring that firefighters are better equipped than ever to protect lives and property.

Man's Quest for Fire. Another Man's Quest To Prevent It From Getting Out of Control

Fire has played an important role in human societies since prehistoric times. In addition to being used for warmth and cooking, fire was also used for ceremonial and religious purposes.

However, fire was also a significant risk to early human communities, as it could quickly spread and destroy entire villages. As a result, early societies developed basic techniques to control and contain fires.

One of the earliest methods of fire prevention was the construction of fireproof structures. In ancient China, buildings were constructed with brick walls and earthen floors, which helped to prevent fires from spreading. In Europe, stone buildings were constructed in the Middle Ages to reduce the risk of fires.

Another important development was the creation of firebreaks. In ancient Greece, for example, soldiers were stationed around cities to create firebreaks by cutting down trees and other vegetation. These firebreaks were designed to prevent fires from spreading by creating gaps in the landscape that fires could not cross.

In addition to these preventative measures, early societies also developed methods of firefighting. As mentioned earlier, they used tools such as buckets, jars, and axes to contain and extinguish fires. Water was also used to fight fires, and early societies developed their own techniques for delivering water to the site of the fire.

Overall, the early history of firefighting is closely linked to the role of fire in human societies. Early communities developed techniques to prevent and control fires, laying the foundation for future developments in firefighting technology and techniques.

Firefighting was a significant concern in ancient Rome, where fires were a common occurrence due to the crowded and densely packed nature of the city. To combat this problem, the Romans developed advanced firefighting techniques and organizations.

One of the most important developments was the establishment of the Vigiles in the 1st century AD. This firefighting brigade was made up of around 7,000 men who were responsible for maintaining order in the city and fighting fires. They were divided into seven cohorts, each with its own responsibilities. One cohort was responsible for firefighting, while others were responsible for enforcing building codes and ensuring that the city's water supply was maintained.

The Vigiles were equipped with advanced firefighting tools, including hand-operated pumps, which were used to draw water from nearby sources and spray it onto fires. They also used hooks, ladders, and axes to contain and extinguish fires.

The Romans also developed advanced water delivery systems, including aqueducts and fountains, which were used to supply water to the city's firefighting brigades. The city was divided into 14 regions, each of which had its own water supply and firefighting equipment.

Despite these advancements, firefighting in ancient Rome was still a dangerous and difficult task. Fires were a constant threat, and the crowded nature of the city made it difficult for firefighters to reach the site of the fire in a timely manner. Nonetheless, the Vigiles played an important role in maintaining order and preventing the spread of fires in ancient Rome.

Firefighting was also an important concern in ancient Greece, where communities developed their own techniques for fighting fires.

One of the most important developments was the creation of the syringe, which was used to pump water from a container and spray it on flames. This device was often made of bronze or copper and was operated by one or more people.

In addition to the syringe, the Greeks also developed a water-delivery system that used pipes to carry water from nearby sources to where it was needed most. This system was used to supply water to public buildings, such as temples and civic buildings, as well as private homes.

The Greeks also used a variety of tools to fight fires, including buckets, axes, and hooks. They also used blankets to smother small fires and prevent them from spreading.

One of the most famous examples of firefighting in ancient Greece was the Battle of Thermopylae in 480 BC, where the Greek army used fire as a weapon against the invading Persian army. The Greeks set fire to the brush and trees around the narrow pass where the battle took place, creating a wall of flames that prevented the Persians from advancing.

Overall, firefighting in ancient Greece was characterized by a combination of advanced technology and practical techniques. The Greeks developed sophisticated water-delivery systems and firefighting tools, while also relying on basic methods such as buckets and blankets to fight fires.

Firefighting was a significant concern in ancient Egypt, where fires could easily spread and cause extensive damage to the city's buildings and infrastructure.

To combat this problem, the ancient Egyptians developed several techniques for fighting fires. One of the most important was the use of clay pots filled with water, which were used to extinguish small fires. These pots were often kept in strategic locations around the city and could be quickly deployed to put out fires.

The ancient Egyptians also used hand-operated pumps, which were used to draw water from wells and pools. These pumps were often operated by multiple people and were used to supply water to the city's firefighting brigades.

In addition to these techniques, the ancient Egyptians also developed a type of fire extinguisher made of clay pots filled with a mixture of water, salt, and vinegar. These pots could be thrown onto small fires to smother them and prevent them from spreading.

Despite these techniques, firefighting in ancient Egypt was still a difficult and dangerous task. Fires could easily spread due to the use of highly flammable materials in the city's buildings, and the limited availability of water made it difficult to extinguish large fires.

Nonetheless, the ancient Egyptians laid the foundation for future developments in firefighting technology and techniques. Their use of water and clay pots as firefighting tools, in particular, would be adapted and improved upon by later civilizations.

Firefighting was also an important concern in ancient China, where communities developed their own techniques for fighting fires.

One of the most significant developments was the use of gunpowder and explosives to create firebreaks. During the Han dynasty (206 BC – 220 AD), the Chinese military began using gunpowder and explosives to create gaps in the landscape that fires could not cross. This technique was also used to create firebreaks around important buildings and other structures.

The ancient Chinese also developed a variety of tools to fight fires, including bamboo ladders and buckets of water. These tools were often used to fight fires in wooden buildings, which were common in China at the time.

In addition to these techniques, the ancient Chinese also developed advanced water-delivery systems, including a system of underground pipes that was used to supply water to the city's firefighting brigades.

Despite these advancements, firefighting in ancient China was still a difficult and dangerous task. Fires could easily spread due to the use of highly flammable materials in the city's buildings, and the limited availability of water made it difficult to extinguish large fires.

Nonetheless, the ancient Chinese laid the foundation for future developments in firefighting technology and techniques. Their use of gunpowder and explosives to create firebreaks, in particular, would be adapted and improved upon by later civilizations.

Firefighting in the Middle Ages

During the Middle Ages, the growth of cities led to an increase in the number of urban fires. Wooden buildings and thatched roofs were common in medieval cities, and the use of open flames for cooking and heating posed a constant threat of fire.

Fires in medieval cities were often catastrophic, as the buildings were closely packed together and the narrow streets made it difficult for firefighters to access the site of the fire. Furthermore, most medieval cities lacked a dedicated firefighting force, relying instead on ad-hoc groups of volunteers and citizens to put out fires.

As a result, fires in medieval cities often caused significant damage and loss of life. The Great Fire of London in 1666, for example, destroyed over 13,000 buildings and left over 100,000 people homeless.

During the Middle Ages, firefighting was largely the responsibility of guilds and religious orders. These groups provided firefighting services to their respective communities and were often the first line of defense against fires.

Guilds, which were associations of craftsmen and merchants, often had a civic responsibility to protect the communities in which they operated. Many guilds established their own firefighting companies and were responsible for maintaining firefighting equipment and training volunteers to fight fires.

Religious orders also played an important role in firefighting during the Middle Ages. Monasteries and convents often had their own firefighting brigades, which were made up of monks and nuns who were trained in firefighting techniques. These brigades were often the only firefighting force in rural areas, where communities were too small to support a dedicated firefighting force.

Despite the important role that guilds and religious orders played in firefighting during the Middle Ages, their efforts were often hampered by a lack of resources and coordination. Fires were still a significant threat, and communities often struggled to mount an effective response. Nonetheless, the efforts of these groups laid the foundation for future developments in firefighting technology and techniques.

Water was a critical tool in medieval firefighting, and communities developed a variety of techniques for delivering water to the site of the fire.

One of the most common techniques was the use of bucket brigades. Volunteers would form a line from the nearest water source to the site of the fire, passing buckets of water along the line to be thrown onto the flames. This technique was effective for small fires, but was less effective for larger fires, where a larger amount of water was needed.

To address this problem, medieval communities developed more sophisticated water delivery systems. In some cities, water was stored in cisterns or reservoirs, which were connected to a network of pipes that carried water to various parts of the city. In other cities, water was delivered by a system of canals or aqueducts.

In some cases, these water delivery systems were operated by private companies, which were responsible for maintaining the infrastructure and ensuring that water was delivered in a timely manner. These companies were often funded by wealthy citizens or the government, and were an important part of the city's firefighting infrastructure.

Overall, water delivery systems were critical to medieval firefighting. Without a reliable source of water, firefighters were unable to effectively fight fires, and communities were left vulnerable to the destructive power of flames.

In addition to bucket brigades and water delivery systems, medieval firefighters also used hand pumps to draw water from nearby sources and spray it onto fires.

Hand pumps were first developed in the 16th century and were a significant improvement over earlier firefighting tools. They were made of wood or metal and could be operated by several people at once. The pumps used suction to draw water from nearby sources and sprayed it onto the fire through a hose or nozzle.

Hand pumps were more effective than bucket brigades, as they allowed firefighters to deliver a larger volume of water to the site of the fire. They were also more portable than water delivery systems, making them easier to use in areas where water was not readily available.

However, hand pumps had their own limitations. They required a significant amount of manpower to operate, and were often difficult to use in crowded or narrow streets. Nonetheless, they were an important development in the history of firefighting and paved the way for future developments in firefighting technology.

In the 17th century, the first fire insurance companies were established in Europe. These companies provided fire insurance to homeowners and businesses, offering financial protection in the event of a fire.

The first fire Insurance company was established in London in 1680, and was followed by other companies throughout Europe. These companies worked by pooling the risk of fire among a large number of policyholders, making it possible to offer affordable fire insurance to individuals and businesses.

Fire insurance was an important development in the history of firefighting, as it provided a financial incentive for individuals and businesses to invest in fire prevention and safety measures. Insurance companies would often inspect buildings before offering insurance, ensuring that they were built to fire safety standards and had adequate firefighting equipment on hand.

While fire insurance did not directly improve firefighting techniques, it played an important role in reducing the risk of fires and promoting fire safety. The development of fire insurance was a significant step forward in the history of firefighting, and helped to lay the foundation for future developments in fire prevention and safety.

Birth of the Engine

In the 18th century, a new type of firefighting tool was developed: the Newsham fire engine. This steam-powered pump was developed by John Smeaton and was named after its inventor, John Newsham.

The Newsham fire engine was a significant improvement over earlier firefighting tools, as it was capable of delivering a much larger volume of water to the site of the fire. It was powered by a steam engine, which drove a pump that could deliver up to 160 gallons of water per minute.

The Newsham fire engine was also more portable than earlier firefighting tools, as it could be mounted on wheels and pulled by horses. This made it easier to use in crowded or narrow streets and allowed firefighters to quickly respond to fires in different parts of the city.

The Newsham fire engine was a significant development in the history of firefighting, as it marked the first use of steam power in firefighting technology. It paved the way for future developments in firefighting tools and equipment, including the use of motorized vehicles and high-pressure water pumps.

The Philadelphia Contributionship, founded in 1752, was one of the first fire insurance companies in the

United States. It was established by Benjamin Franklin and a group of other civic-minded citizens in response to the frequent fires that occurred in Philadelphia at the time.

The Contributionship worked by pooling the risk of fire among a group of policyholders, offering financial protection in the event of a fire. It also played an important role in promoting fire safety and prevention, conducting inspections of buildings and offering advice on fire prevention measures.

The Contributionship was an important development in the history of firefighting in the United States, as it helped to promote fire safety and provided financial protection to individuals and businesses. It was also a model for future fire insurance companies, many of which were established in other cities across the United States.

Today, the Contributionship is still in operation, offering fire insurance and promoting fire safety and prevention in the Philadelphia area. It is the oldest insurance company in the United States and a testament to the enduring legacy of Benjamin Franklin's civic-minded spirit.

In the 19th century, the first firefighting academies were established in Europe and North America. These academies provided formal training in firefighting techniques and equipment, helping to professionalize the firefighting profession.

The first firefighting academy was established in Berlin in 1854, followed by similar academies in other European cities. In North America, the first firefighting academy was established in Cincinnati in 1874, followed by other academies in cities such as Chicago and New York.

Firefighting academies provided a structured curriculum that covered a wide range of topics, including fire behavior, firefighting tactics, and the use of firefighting equipment. Students were also trained in physical fitness and endurance, as firefighting was a physically demanding profession.

The establishment of firefighting academies helped to professionalize the firefighting profession and improve the effectiveness of firefighting efforts. Firefighters were better equipped to handle fires and were able to work more efficiently as a team.

Today, firefighting academies continue to provide training and education to firefighters around the world. They are an important part of the firefighting profession, helping to ensure that firefighters are well-trained and prepared to respond to emergencies.

In the early 20th century, motorized firefighting equipment began to replace traditional horse-drawn equipment. This shift marked a significant improvement in the speed and efficiency of firefighting efforts.

The first motorized fire engines were introduced in the United States in the early 1900s, and were quickly adopted by fire departments across the country. These engines were powered by internal combustion engines, which allowed them to travel at much faster speeds than horse-drawn engines.

Motorized fire engines were also equipped with more advanced firefighting equipment, including high-pressure water pumps and hoses that could deliver water to the site of the fire from greater distances.

The Introduction of motorized firefighting equipment was a significant development in the history of firefighting, as it marked a shift towards more advanced and efficient firefighting techniques. It allowed firefighters to respond to emergencies more quickly and effectively, reducing the risk of damage and loss of life.

Today, motorized firefighting equipment is standard in fire

departments around the world. It continues to be improved and refined, with new technologies and equipment being developed to improve the effectiveness of firefighting efforts.

In the modern era, fire prevention education has become an important part of firefighting efforts. Fire prevention education programs are designed to raise awareness about fire safety and prevention, helping to reduce the risk of fires and promote fire safety in homes, schools, and businesses.

Fire prevention education programs cover a wide range of topics, including the importance of smoke detectors, the dangers of electrical fires, and the proper use of flammable materials. They also provide information on how to create a fire escape plan, and what to do in the event of a fire.

Fire prevention education is an important part of the firefighting profession, as it helps to reduce the risk of fires and prevent loss of life and property damage. By educating the public about fire safety and prevention, firefighters are able to promote a culture of safety and preparedness that can help to prevent fires before they occur.

Today, fire prevention education programs are offered in schools, community centers, and other public venues. They continue to be an important part of the firefighting profession, helping to promote fire safety and prevent fires in communities around the world.

Evolving Techniques and Technology

In the early modern period, firefighting technology continued to evolve, with new tools and equipment being developed to help firefighters respond to emergencies more effectively.

One of the most important developments in firefighting technology was the introduction of steam-powered fire engines. These engines were first developed in the early 19th century and were capable of delivering large amounts of water to the site of a fire, helping to extinguish flames more quickly and effectively.

Steam-powered fire engines were also equipped with hoses and nozzles that could be used to direct water onto the fire, making them more versatile than earlier firefighting tools. They were often mounted on wheels and could be pulled by horses, making them more portable than earlier engines.

Another important development in firefighting technology was the introduction of fire hydrants. Hydrants were first introduced in the mid-19th

century and allowed firefighters to tap into the city's water supply to extinguish fires. They were often connected to a network of pipes that carried water throughout the city, making it easier for firefighters to access water when they needed it.

Overall, the evolution of firefighting technology in the early modern period was a significant development in the history of firefighting. It allowed firefighters to respond to emergencies more effectively and efficiently, reducing the risk of damage and loss of life. The development of new tools and equipment would continue to play an important role in the firefighting profession, paving the way for future advancements in firefighting technology.

The Industrial Revolution, which occurred in the 18th and 19th centuries, had a significant impact on the development of firefighting technology. The growth of industry led to an increase in the number of fires, as factories and mills often contained large amounts of flammable materials.

To address this challenge, new firefighting tools and equipment were developed, including steam-powered fire engines and high-pressure water pumps. These innovations were made possible by the technological advancements of the Industrial

Revolution, which allowed for the development of more powerful engines and pumps.

In addition to new tools and equipment, the Industrial Revolution also led to the creation of new firefighting organizations. Professional firefighting departments were established in many cities, staffed by paid firefighters who were trained in the use of new firefighting technology.

The Industrial Revolution also had an impact on building design, as architects began to incorporate fire safety features into their designs. Buildings were constructed of more fire-resistant materials, such as brick and stone, and fire escapes and sprinkler systems were installed to help prevent fires and facilitate evacuations.

The Industrial Revolution played a significant role in the development of firefighting technology and organizations. It led to the creation of new tools and equipment, and promoted the professionalization of the firefighting profession. It also helped to promote fire safety and prevention, laying the foundation for future advancements in fire prevention and safety.

In the early modern period, professional fire departments began to emerge in many cities around the world. These departments were staffed by paid firefighters who were trained in the use of new firefighting tools and equipment, and were dedicated to responding to emergencies quickly and efficiently.

One of the first professional fire departments was established in Edinburgh, Scotland in 1824. The Edinburgh Fire Brigade was staffed by paid firefighters who were equipped with steam-powered fire engines and other firefighting tools. Similar departments were established in other cities, including London, Paris, and New York.

Professional fire departments were a significant development in the history of firefighting, as they allowed for a more coordinated and effective response to emergencies. Firefighters were able to work together as a team, using their specialized skills and training to extinguish fires and protect lives and property.

Professional fire departments also helped to promote the professionalization of the firefighting profession, raising the standards for training and equipment and helping to create a more respected and prestigious profession.

Today, professional fire departments continue to be an important part of the firefighting profession. They are staffed by highly trained firefighters who are equipped with the latest firefighting technology.

Humor on the Job

While firefighting is a serious and often dangerous profession, humor has long played an important role in firefighting culture. From funny stories and jokes shared around the station to the lighthearted pranks and good-natured ribbing that are common among firefighters, humor can help to build camaraderie, relieve stress, and foster a sense of community among firefighters.

Despite the serious nature of their work, firefighters often use humor as a coping mechanism, helping them to maintain a positive attitude and stay focused even in the face of difficult or traumatic situations. Whether it's a funny story shared after a long shift or a well-timed joke to break the tension during a tense situation, humor can be a powerful tool for firefighters, helping them to stay mentally and emotionally resilient in the face of adversity.

Overall, the role of humor in firefighting culture reflects the unique challenges and stresses of the profession, as well as the close bonds and sense of community that exist among firefighters. By finding ways to laugh and stay positive even in difficult situations, firefighters are able to maintain a sense of perspective and stay focused on their critical mission of protecting their communities from harm.

One of the most important benefits of humor in firefighting is its role in promoting positive mental health and well-being among firefighters. The high-stress nature of firefighting can take a toll on the mental and emotional health of firefighters, leading to anxiety, depression, and other mental health issues. However, humor can help to reduce these negative effects by promoting feelings of happiness, relaxation, and social connectedness.

Studies have shown that laughter and humor can promote the release of endorphins and other "feel-good" chemicals in the brain, reducing stress and promoting feelings of well-being. This can be especially important for firefighters, who are often exposed to traumatic events and high-stress situations that can cause long-term emotional and psychological effects.

There are numerous funny anecdotes in the daily life of a firefighter. These stories may be completely true, somewhat embellished, or as tall as the tales lumberjacks used to tell about Paul Bunyan. This is a collection of just a few:

A group of firefighters responded to a call about a fire in a large office building. When they arrived on the scene, they found that the fire was on the top floor of the building, and the only way to get there was through a narrow staircase.

As they made their way up the staircase, they quickly realized that the stairwell was filled with smoke and that visibility was extremely limited. One firefighter suggested that they hold onto each other's belts to stay together and avoid getting separated.

As they continued up the stairs, one firefighter suddenly yelled out, "I think we're going the wrong way!" The others were confused and asked him how he knew. "Because the fire's getting bigger," he replied. The group quickly turned around and made their way back down the stairs, thankful for their sense of humor and quick thinking in a challenging situation.

The Rookie's First Call

When a rookie firefighter responded to his first emergency call, he was determined to prove himself as a capable and competent member of the team. However, when he arrived on the scene and saw the flames leaping out of a burning building, he froze in fear.

Thankfully, one of the senior firefighters quickly took charge, guiding the rookie through the process of setting up the hoses and dousing the flames. Afterwards, the senior firefighter gave the rookie a pat on the back and said, "Don't worry, kid. We all freeze up on our first call. The important thing is that you kept your cool and did your job."

The Cat In the Tree

One day, the fire department received a call about a cat that was stuck in a tree. Although the firefighters knew that this was not a true emergency, they decided to respond to the call anyway, eager to help the feline in distress.

When they arrived on the scene, they found the cat perched high up in a tree, mewing pitifully. The firefighters tried coaxing the cat down with treats and toys, but nothing seemed to work.

Finally, one of the firefighters had an idea. He put on a pair of thick gloves, climbed up the tree, and reached out to the cat. To his surprise, the cat immediately climbed onto his shoulder and nuzzled against his neck.

The firefighters were overjoyed to have rescued the cat, and took turns holding and petting it as they drove it to the local animal shelter.

The Old Firehouse

One of the oldest firehouses in town was scheduled to be torn down and replaced with a new, modern facility. However, before the demolition crews arrived, the firefighters decided to hold a farewell party for the old firehouse.

As the firefighters reminisced about all of the calls they had responded to over the years, they began to hear strange noises coming from the walls. It soon became clear that a family of raccoons had taken up residence in the firehouse, and were protesting the impending demolition.

Despite the challenges of evicting the raccoons, the firefighters were determined to do so without harming them. After several hours of coaxing and negotiating, they were finally able to persuade the raccoons to leave, and the demolition proceeded as planned. However, the firefighters would always remember the raccoons as a memorable part of the history of their beloved old firehouse.

The Thanksgiving Turkey

One Thanksgiving Day, a family was roasting a turkey in their oven when suddenly, flames began to shoot out from the stove. Panicked, the family called 911 and within minutes, a group of firefighters arrived on the scene.

Despite the chaos and confusion of the situation, one of the firefighters noticed that the turkey in the oven was still cooking, and suggested that they should try to save it if possible. The firefighters carefully removed the turkey from the oven and carried it outside to safety, much to the family's delight and relief.

Although the family's Thanksgiving meal was disrupted by the unexpected emergency, they would always be grateful to the firefighters who went above and beyond to save not only their home, but their holiday dinner as well.

The Ladder Race

One year, two rival firehouses decided to hold a friendly competition to see who could raise their ladder the fastest. The two teams set up their ladders side by side, and at the signal, they began to raise them up towards the sky.

As the ladders climbed higher and higher, the two teams matched each other move for move, neither one gaining a clear advantage. However, as they reached the top of the ladders, one of the firefighters suddenly lost his footing and began to fall towards the ground.

Quickly, the other firefighters sprang into action, catching their teammate and lowering him safely back to the ground. Although they had lost the ladder race, the firefighters knew that they had won something much more important – the trust and respect of their fellow firefighters.

The Flooded Basement

One rainy night, a family woke up to find that their basement was flooded with water. Desperate for help, they called the fire department and within minutes, a team of firefighters arrived on the scene.

Despite the late hour and the soggy conditions, the firefighters worked tirelessly to pump out the water and dry out the basement. As they worked, they chatted with the family and made jokes to keep their spirits up.

By the time they were finished, the basement was dry and the family was smiling again. The firefighters, too, were pleased to have made a difference in the lives of their community members, even in the midst of a challenging and unexpected situation.

The Birthday Surprise

One day, a group of firefighters received a special request from a family in their community. It was their son's fifth birthday, and all he wanted was to ride in a fire truck.

Without hesitation, the firefighters arranged to surprise the young boy with a ride in the fire truck, complete with lights and sirens. As they drove through the streets of the neighborhood, the boy beamed with excitement and joy.

At the end of the ride, the firefighters presented the boy with a special firefighter hat and badge, making him an honorary firefighter for the day. The family was deeply grateful for the firefighters' kindness and generosity, and the young boy would always remember his unforgettable fifth birthday.

The Cat Rescue

One day, a family's beloved pet cat became trapped high up in a tree, unable to climb down. Despite the family's best efforts to coax the cat down, it remained stuck in the tree for hours.

Finally, the family called the fire department for help. Within minutes, a group of firefighters arrived on the scene and quickly assessed the situation.

Using a tall ladder and a bucket truck, the firefighters were able to reach the cat and bring it down safely to the ground. The family was overjoyed to be reunited with their beloved pet, and the firefighters were pleased to have been able to make a difference in the lives of both the cat and its grateful family.

The Fire Drill

One day, a group of firefighters decided to hold a surprise fire drill for the residents of a local nursing home. The drill involved evacuating the residents from their rooms and guiding them to safety, simulating a real emergency situation.

As they worked, the firefighters were struck by the courage and resilience of the elderly residents, many of whom had physical disabilities or memory loss. Despite the chaos and confusion of the drill, the residents remained calm and cooperative, trusting the firefighters to guide them to safety.

After the drill was over, the firefighters were greeted with hugs and words of thanks from the grateful residents. It was a reminder of the importance of their work, and the impact they could have on the lives of their community members, especially those who were most vulnerable.

The Stuck Dog

One day, a family's dog became trapped in a small drainage pipe in their backyard, unable to get out. The family tried everything they could think of to free the dog, but it remained stuck.

Finally, the family called the fire department for help. A group of firefighters arrived on the scene and quickly assessed the situation. Using their training and expertise, they carefully and gently pulled the dog out of the pipe and reunited it with its grateful family.

The family was overjoyed to have their beloved pet back safe and sound, and the firefighters were pleased to have been able to make a difference in the life of both the dog and its family.

The Thanksgiving Food Drive

One year, a group of firefighters decided to hold a Thanksgiving food drive for families in need in their community. They collected donations of food and money from local businesses and community members, and then set out to deliver the food baskets to families in their area.

As they went from house to house, the firefighters were touched by the gratitude and appreciation of the families they visited. For many of them, the food baskets would mean the difference between a meager or non-existent Thanksgiving meal and a bountiful feast with loved ones.

The firefighters felt proud and humbled to have been able to make a difference in the lives of their community members, especially during the holiday season.

The Water Main Break

One day, a large water main broke in a busy downtown area, causing flooding and chaos on the streets. The fire department was called in to help, and they quickly got to work pumping water out of the flooded areas and directing traffic.

As they worked, the firefighters were struck by the bravery and resilience of the nearby business owners and workers, who worked tirelessly to mitigate the damage and keep their businesses running despite the unexpected setback.

The firefighters worked hard to ensure the safety and well-being of everyone in the area, and were pleased to be able to make a difference in the lives of those affected by the water main break. It was a reminder of the importance of teamwork and community in the face of unexpected challenges.

The Surprise Visit

One day, a group of firefighters decided to pay a surprise visit to a local children's hospital. Dressed in their full firefighter gear, they visited the patients in their rooms, handing out firefighter hats and stickers and sharing stories and jokes with the children.

The children were thrilled to meet the firefighters and to learn more about their work, and the firefighters were touched by the resilience and bravery of the young patients they met. It was a reminder of the importance of bringing joy and light to those who were going through difficult times.

The Stranded Motorist

One day, a motorist became stranded on the side of a busy highway, with a flat tire and no spare. As cars whizzed past, the driver felt helpless and alone.

Luckily, a group of firefighters happened to be driving by and noticed the stranded motorist. They pulled over and quickly got to work changing the tire, using their expertise and teamwork to get the job done quickly and safely.

The stranded motorist was grateful for the firefighters' help and kindness, and the firefighters were pleased to have been able to make a difference in the life of someone in need.

The Unexpected Fire

One day, a small fire broke out in a residential neighborhood, catching everyone by surprise. As smoke billowed from the house, neighbors rushed to call the fire department, who arrived on the scene quickly and efficiently.

Despite the unexpectedness of the fire, the firefighters were able to contain it quickly and prevent it from spreading to nearby homes. They worked tirelessly to ensure the safety of everyone in the area, and were able to put out the fire completely within a matter of hours.

The homeowners were grateful for the firefighters' quick response and bravery, and the firefighters felt proud and humbled to have been able to make a difference in the lives of those affected by the fire. It was a reminder of the importance of being prepared and ready for anything, no matter how unexpected.

Stories like these are an integral part of firefighter culture because they help to shape the collective identity and values of the firefighting community. By sharing stories of bravery, sacrifice, and service, firefighters reinforce the importance of these values and create a sense of shared purpose and mission.

Moreover, stories can be a source of inspiration and motivation for firefighters, reminding them of the importance of their work and of the impact they have on their communities. These stories can also serve as a way of recognizing and honoring the sacrifices and contributions of firefighters, both past and present.

Stories can also help to build camaraderie and solidarity among firefighters, who often form close bonds through shared experiences and challenges. By sharing stories with one another, firefighters can create a sense of shared history and culture, and can build trust and respect within their teams.

Finally, stories can be a way of passing on knowledge and expertise from one generation of firefighters to the next. By sharing their experiences and insights, veteran firefighters can help to train and mentor new recruits, and can ensure that the traditions and best practices of firefighting are preserved and passed down.

In all of these ways, stories play a vital role in shaping the culture and identity of the firefighting community, and in honoring the bravery, sacrifice, and service of those who dedicate their lives to protecting their communities from fire and other dangers.

In Honor

Firefighters are more than just first responders. They are heroes, guardians, and protectors of our communities. They embody the very essence of bravery and selflessness, putting their lives on the line each day to protect us from the dangers of fire and other emergencies.

Their dedication and sacrifice inspire us all to be better people, to stand up for what is right, and to put the needs of others before our own. Firefighters are the unsung heroes of our society, working tirelessly behind the scenes to keep us safe, often at great personal risk.

As we go about our daily lives, we can rest assured that there are brave men and women out there, always ready to answer the call when danger strikes. They are the firefighters, and we owe them a debt of gratitude that can never be fully repaid.

There is something truly awe-inspiring about firefighters. Maybe it's the way they rush into burning buildings without hesitation, or the way they work together seamlessly as a team to fight the flames. Or maybe it's the way they always seem to have a smile or a kind word, even in the face of danger and adversity.

Whatever it is, firefighters have a special place in our hearts. They are the embodiment of courage, resilience, and compassion, always ready to lend a helping hand to those in need. They are the protectors of our homes, businesses, and communities, and we are forever grateful for their service and sacrifice.

We must never forget the bravery and dedication of our firefighters, nor the sacrifices they make every day to keep us safe. They are our heroes, our role models, and our friends, and we are honored to have them in our lives. They are the very definition of selflessness and service, and we owe them a debt of gratitude that can never be fully repaid.

When we think about firefighters, words like bravery, heroism, and sacrifice come to mind. These men and women are the true guardians of our communities, working tirelessly to keep us safe from the dangers of fire and other emergencies.

We often take for granted the risks that firefighters face on a daily basis, putting their own lives on the line to protect ours. We forget that they are husbands, wives, mothers, fathers, sons, and daughters who leave their loved ones at home each day to serve their communities.

Yet, despite the dangers they face, firefighters remain committed to their mission, always ready to answer the call when duty calls. They are the epitome of bravery and selflessness, and their dedication to serving others is an inspiration to us all.

As we go about our daily lives, let us remember the sacrifices and contributions of our firefighters, and let us honor them by living up to their example of service, compassion, and bravery. We owe them a debt of gratitude that can never be fully repaid, but we can show our appreciation by supporting them, thanking them, and always remembering the heroic work that they do.

www.ingramcontent.com/pod-product-compliance
Lightning Source LLC
Chambersburg PA
CBHW070611220526
45467CB00003B/1373